The Three Commandments of Eating

By

Dr. Wayne Pickering N.D., Th.D., Sc.M.

Copyright © 2011 by The Center for Nutrition.

This is the Transcripts of a Live Seminar from Dr. Wayne's "Is Your Diet A Riot" DVD Series.

This portion of this series is all about the combining of our foods. OK. How do we mix foods to where we get the most out of it? To where we don't have to worry about all these hassles of digestion. I mean you look down at the rows and the rows in the grocery stores, health food stores, everything, where you got digestive aids, indigestion remedies, stuff to help make move food through you. Everything that has something to do with digestion.

It's amazing, it's the largest selling niched item in any food store. In any health food store, any chain, you look at any grocery store, and this is it. So there's got to be some emphasis put on since we know now the foods we shouldn't be eating to anything that's white, anything that fizzes, anything that is greasy. If it's white it ain't right. If it fizzes you'll fizzle. And if it's greasy it's sleazy. We don't eat it. So what are the three commandments of eating that we can put together to where everything that I eat stands the best chance of going through me with the least aggravation? What are they?

There are seven proper food combining rules. That's why we put together the Food Combining Guide, but a lot of people did not have room in their home for that size so we decided to go ahead and make the Food Combining Guide post. But it shows you all of the foods and what they are, how to mix them, how long they take to digest, if they are acid or alkaline, when they are in season, and all that. So there's seven proper food combining rules, but there are three commandments you can't deviate from and here is the first one, these three commandments, if you'll abide these three, embrace them, your digestion will pick up immensely.

The first one is this: and it's a little duel thought on this one commandment: Dessert, good desserts, get away from them. Eat them before the meal and never after. And wish you, oh boy, you guy's love me already. Now, so we need to eat the dessert before the meal, never after. Remember a little while ago I shared with you "today we're serving food on the basis of taste and tradition and we do it in haste and we forgot nutrition." OK so we are always doing things traditionally, have the dessert after. If we had it before it would digest. But if we have it after it does not, cannot, will not digest. Bottom line. But if you eat it before, it digests.

So what I want to do is to show you right now what happens to food when we eat. I mean, why does it look so different the second time I get to see it. I mean, there is a certain chain reaction that's going on here. I mean, have you ever thought about it? Why does the banana make skin, or how does it affect the air. How to make teeth. I mean, this juicy thing right here, banana, is going to make skin. It's going to make hair, it's going to make skin, it's going to make teeth, it's going to make eyes, ears. Dates, choose medjool dates, delicious, right off the bat. All that stuff is going to go from this to this. That is interesting to me. I said how does that happen anyway?

So if you will take a look at the body and understand how the body works, and get away from all of the hype, and all of the things that are being touted as the elixir, the best. If we can get away from that and understand how this body works, then we don't have any confusion about what we need to eat. The whole ticket is to get you to want to do it. You see, you already know how to eat. You know how to do that. I don't have to teach you how to eat. All I have to do is just change the stuff. Because you're already doing that. You see?

You just have to change. Sometimes we give in and we stay with the problems that we have rather than give in to the uncertainty of change. Nobody like change except a wet baby (paraphrasing a good friend of mine, Joe Marino). Nobody likes change except a wet baby. We resist it. We don't want it. Whatever. So sometimes we endure unhappy marriages, hate our jobs, because of the uncertainty of change. We don't like to take a swing at the ball a lot of times, do you see? Scared we might strike out. So I think that if we will understand the way this body works and embrace the principles and then try this. Try this. Try this. Try this. Nobody does things right.

Notice when we were in school we learned that two plus two equals four. Two times two equals four. Three times three is nine. Three plus three equal six. And when we got that down then we knew how to divide. And then we knew how to subtract, and all that. So we have to learn little steps. What I'm doing here with you right now is we're laying out how this whole thing works and then I want you, with your schedule, pick out a few things that you like, make that a habit, and then go to the next level.

A high jumper never starts at six feet, he starts at five feet. Then he goes to five-one. And when he is comfortable there he goes to five-two. And right up the line. Don't you agree?

So if we will take little things, bit by bit, piece by piece, and adjust it to our schedule, and then after a while he goes, "Boy this is delicious." The young fellow that was helping me today said, "I hate dates." I said, "have you had one?" "No," I said, "how do you know you hate them if you never had them?" So I gave it to him and he goes, "Mmmm. This is good." Which is the universal language by the way.

When I was in Viet Nam, I never will forget a little side story. In Viet Nam, I remember there's an old Papasaun, he had tattoos from his nose to his toes. And that guy put every tattoo on his body. I mean he had one tooth, hanging out the side of his mouth, couldn't speak any English, and he was going on with his Vietnamese, and I had this little mango, it was a great mango. And I'm sitting over there under this palm tree, just cutting this mango open a little bit, see, way off down there in the Mekong Delta, I'll never forget, a little town called Vin Long. On the outskirts of Vin Long, and Vin Long is the outskirts.

So here I was way up in the sticks, and I was cutting this mango open and, under this palm tree, and this old Papasaun, had a little plank going all the way down his little hooch out there on four sticks in the mud, and he walked over there, and he was staring at me, had great bit old baggy pants on him, just looking like this. He was looking at me, I knew he wanted some of that mango. Now I couldn't speak Vietnamese too well, I could speak it pretty good now, but I couldn't at the time. And he couldn't speak a word of English, except number 10, number 1. And so I was eating this mango and I gave him a little of the mango. I said "Papasaun, here, would you like?" "Mmmm, OK, OK." He could say OK. So I gave him a mango. And do you know what the universal language is? <u>Mmmmmmm.</u> But, you knew that sound. Just like that young kid with those dates, loved it right off the bat. I didn't have to bribe him. It was just one of those things we just love anyway.

So, what I want to do is to take you on a little journey and this right now is the single greatest lesson I can teach you about this portion of today. On this portion of this seminar series right now, this is the single greatest lesson that you can start learning about your body right now is that we all digest food exactly the same way. You prove me wrong, I will buy you the dream home of your choice, pay off your car, buy anything that you want, and take you on a year's vacation to wherever you want, down to Bora Bora, if you want. It's yours.

I have invited any physician because I'm approved for continuing education by the Florida and Alabama Boards of Pharmacy, anything that you hear from me that you can take into the bank, or just recently a approved for continuing education by the Florida Board of Dentistry, that every time that a Dentist in Florida or a

Pharmacist in Florida and Alabama hear me speak, they get continuing education credits for their license again for another year. And everything that I am teaching is the antitheses of the protocol of pharmacology. The direct opposite is a hoot. But the point being that none of them has ever accepted my challenge about – we all digest food exactly the same way. I said, you prove me wrong.

And let me extend that just a little bit. If you look at the way we work, this first of all is the way we look. This is the digestive system. This is how we look. Ok. You take a look at any textbook on physiology and anatomy and never once does it say Wayne Pickering up there, Ron Drake, never does say that, doesn't say any of you guys' name in there at all, does it?

Doesn't say that. Doesn't say Michael Stahl, it doesn't say Rosita Perez, it doesn't say Wayne Pickering. It says, in the mouth we do it this way. In the stomach we do it this way. In the duodenum we do it this way. We all digest food exactly the same way. Our rate of efficiency of the breakdown may vary, and our needs may vary. You may be sitting behind the desk as a graphic artist and I could be a Triathlete. Our needs may vary but the way we do it is identical. Good news. We are species specific. If you put horses in Africa, you put them in China, you put them in the United States, Canada, wherever you put them, they are going to digest food exactly the same way. They are species specific. We are humans. We are species specific. We have a certain digestive track that is irrefutable, exactly the same. Sometimes we get butchered up in the operating table, and some of it is cut out of his or whatever because of cancer or what have you. But we do it the same. If you will embrace that, now we can move forward.

All right, how does food digest? Let's go over to this chart over here. Food in the mouth, it comes down this way here, comes down through here. Now in this portion up here, over here, down here, and out the rectum. So there is thirty feet from here to here. What happens in the process?

First of all, there are four processes the body employs. By the way, I'm going to teach you the best lesson you've ever learned about nutrition. Nutrition doesn't heal, it doesn't cure, vitamins don't heal, and vitamins don't cure.

Nothing heals or cures except the body. And when you lay out the foundation for health, your body will do its best job of healing as a result. So if you're having a problem, stop causing the problem, embrace all of the elements of health, and watch your body do some phenomenal things. I mean from the worst conditions, you'd be amazed. Nothing more, there's nothing more, there's nothing magical about it, there's nothing mysterious about it. All nutrition is is a series of four processes. Four. That the body employs to make food so what happens to food in the process?

First of all there are four, now here's nutrition. Nutrition is materials for the body to use. That's all. That's all nutrition is. A series of four processes the body employs to make food materials for the body to use. Hence, that's where we come up with the saying "If you want to be tough, you've got to eat good stuff." All right, now the first process - the body breaks this food down from this to this. So it has to break it down. Now it has to get into the blood stream. Then the body will use it. Then it will eliminate it. Four processes. The body breaks it down, digests, then the body gets it into the blood stream, it's called absorption, then the body will use it, it's called assimilation, then the body eliminates, elimination. Basic physiology. Digestion, Absorption, Assimilation, Elimination.

OK, we don't have any say-so about all of that. If we had to worry about, OK, epiglottis close, we don't want the food going into the lungs. Get through the cardia valve, open up. Now hydrochloric acid, pump. All right now, pyloric valve, open up. Bile secrete so much sodium bicarbonate from the pancreas, get in here, come on out, we need it quick. OK. Now if you had to worry about all that you'd never get anything done. It's all autonomic, innate. It's innate wisdom that governs. You blink twelve times a minute. Your body digests food. You don't need things to enhance digestion. You need to stop hurting digestion and then the body takes over innately, sub-cortically, because that's its natural tendency towards normalcy.

So here are the four places that food breaks down. Because that's all we have any say so about, is where does the food break down. In the mouth - 1, in the stomach - 2, in the duodenum -

3, and this jejunum here - 4. Now I don't want this to go over your head. Because if anybody ever comes in and says "that's not true, wait a minute," it says right here, this is how we work, here's the four places where the food breaks down, this is not the four processes, this is the first process, the breakdown, one, two, three, four.

In the mouth it starts to begin its digestion, in an alkaline digestive juice, very important that we remember these little things. The only food that breaks down chemically – now incidentally, there are two kinds of digestion. You got the mechanical, chewing. Then you got the chemical, saliva, hydrochloric acid, all these different chemicals do you see that it takes to break the food down chemically. And there's only one food that chemically breaks down on the stomach. Just one, protein. And it's always in a very acid state. Now stage one, alkaline. Stage two is acid. Stage three and four are all alkaline.

Now here are the commandments. What was the first one? Desert the desserts. Check out what happens now in the process of the movement through the food. You have a valve here, it's called the cardiac valve, that is actually a sphincter, that opens like this and will allow the food from the esophagus to go into the stomach and then they'll close back. Much like, uh, let me give you an analogy. Let's say your commode. Notice when you flush the commode the refuse goes down, it doesn't come back up, because there is a check valve in there that closes off and doesn't allow it to come back. Don't you agree?

All right that's the same principle that happens here. Notice when you eat something and you throw up, the pain should hurt here where the stuff is coming out. But it doesn't. It always hurts here worst because that sphincter has done something that's not normal, it does a back flip, so to speak, and shoots it up. That's why this pain is so bad here when you vomit.

So, the food will allow it to come in here, now while the food is doing this and this in the stomach it's not going to shoot it back out the mouth. Now you've got one, you'll understand why desert the desserts first, when you understand these two valves. You've got one valve that leaves the stomach. It's called the pyloric valve. It acts like another sphincter, the pyloric valve, will allow the food to come out of the stomach and through into stage three and backs off. So here's where your desserts and all of your sweets digest, right here and here.

What's the only food that chemically digests in the stomach? Protein. And it's in an alkaline state, excuse me acid state. And the alkaline, everything digests along through here, they finish the digestion. But this is alkaline. Well if acids and alkalines neutralize each other, how does that work? You have a component in your pancreas, there's an enzyme called sodium bicarbonate. And it acts like a neutralizer kind of thing that will allow a favorable environment for this to pick up its digestion again. It's like soda ash. You get indigestion and you drink soda ash, baking soda or something like that, it'll neutralize kind of a thing, that's the basic principle there. This is natural. The soda ash is not.

OK Desert the desserts. Why? And here's the true commandment. Eat melons alone or leave them alone or your stomach will moan. Here's the deal. You eat your desserts first. Very little mechanical action is done on those sweets in the stomach. No chemical at all and very little mechanical. But the valve will open and allow that food to come in here and it would back up into the stomach while you are digesting other food. So if you eat the dessert before the meal it will get through these two valves and digestion is OK. It's cool. So then, you eat the dessert, wait thirty minutes, let it get through here, and then you can eat your meal and get away with it. But if you eat it after you're always going to have trouble. You're looking for something for your indigestion. Or you're bound up. Or you're miserable. You're not feeling good. You got terrible gas. Oh, what am I going to do about this? And if you just switch that around, that will be tremendous. Desert the desserts. Eat them before the meal, never after, and eat melons alone or leave them alone, or the stomach will moan. Now why is that? Because melons are very, very simple sugar. They are broken down almost, they are in the simplest form to begin with, and so they'll come right down in here almost immediately with a little bit of digestion here and they'll get in through here and this will work nicely. You eat them after a meal, you'll always have problems…First Commandment.

The Second Commandment, and there's three of them, is don't mix fruits and vegetables at the same meal. Now why is that? OK where do fruits do their digestion? Where do fruits do their digestion? In stage three and four, isn't that correct? Alright. Now the vegetables have a lot of fiber and they take an incredible amount of time in the stomach breaking down, breaking down, breaking down. If the fruit is held back in the stomach digesting all those vegetables and mixing together and everything, you're going to have fermentation. Same, same. The food rotting in your system. And that's part of the reason why indigestion is so prevalent, just because of that one little thing.

And you know I find an awful lot of people, they will go to these salad bars and eat just about everything you can think of. They eat enough cellulose to choke a grazing steer. And they'll come back later on and eat all this melon, and they have mayonnaise on it. And people actually salt this watermelon. I know we all did that. We all did. Hey what do you mean we all did it, honey? We still doing it. But people do that. Isn't that amazing? They actually put poison on this just 'cause the flavor, you see, it's the taste. Alright, so you're probably back there saying, "what's wrong with that?" So, the fruit and the vegetables at the same meal, is not a good deal. It's the second commandment.

But the Third Commandment is really the worst one of all. It's the proteins and the starches. That means the hamburger on the bun. The macaroni and the cheese. The chicken and the rice. The meat and the potatoes. The spaghetti and the meatballs. The macaroni and the cheese. And all of those things that we're eating, we call it it's the standard American diet. It's in sad shape. It's pitiful at best. Why is that? I mean, come on we're hearing a lot about that, but why is that? When we eat starches and proteins, what is the place where starches begin the digestion? In the mouth. Now first of all, how many places is there that food breaks down? There are four. Starches need three places in the body to digest, break down. And it's the only food that needs three stages to break down. So now if there is only one food that chemically breaks down in the stomach, let's use our intelligence here, and rational, if there is only one food that breaks down in the stomach and it's protein, we've only get three places left where other foods digest, don't we? OK. And since starch needs three places to break down, what's the most logically place for starch to begin their digestion. It would be in the mouth, wouldn't it? And it's the only food that breaks down in the mouth with an enzyme here called salivary amylase, or you call it ptyalin, something like that.

That's all in our Food Combining Guide for you if you want to come up and look at it or on that little card that we gave you. So starches begin their digestion in the mouth in an alkaline state. Now when we're eating proteins and starches together, the protein, your body does not want to be poisoned, it does not want to be poisoned, and protein will turn to alcohols. And here's the line. This stuff turns to alcohol and gas. Now your body hates the alcohol and of course your friends hate the gas, you see. But they start their digestion in the mouth, the starch, and then all of a sudden that stops immediately because the protein needs to start digesting in an acid state right away. So now you've got food fermenting in the stomach from the starch and this is coming down. Now you're having turmoil in the stomach pathetically. Now when you finally get down here to stage three and stage four, you've got so much acid and so much bad things going on here you're going to say, "how does it get to the blood stream? How does it get to the adipose tissue? How does it make tissue? If it's so bad? Well, we're getting cancer. We're getting heart disease. We're getting skin problems. We're getting teeth problems. We can't see near as good, you see. And we're getting irritable. We're getting all of those things that is totally not normal.

And age does not cause sickness. Just because you're sixty. Just because you're seventy. You should never, ever, ever be sick. You never catch disease. You earn it. You never catch disease. You earn it. And it stems from crud in the blood from being drunk with junk. If we will understand these truisms then we don't have to be worried about it. Whether it is the want. Do we want it? And the old line goes – people only want what we want, when the want is more than the cost, more than the effort, more than the price we need to pay. OK. People only want what they want, when the want is more than the effort. That's why I want to make this whole thing very simple.

I'm giving quite a bit of technical terms here for you but when you see the simplicity of this, all we have to do now is just embrace a few things and we can get on a roll. OK. So no proteins and starches at the same meal. How many people here planted a garden? Has anybody ever planted a garden? OK. Notice what you had to do with the soil. You had to make sure it balanced. And what we did is we had a nice plot you see, and we took a sample here, a sample here, one in the middle, one in each corner. We took it down to the feed store and they did their test. And it was too alkaline. Well we had to put a little chicken manure on there, because chicken manure is so acidic and it would kind of balance the soil. Alright, now we do it, we till it up and do all the – and somebody said, "Wayne, you buy so many vegetables why don't you just grow them." I said," I did, I don't want to do that anymore. You can grow them; I'll buy them from you."

So we'll take it back down to the feed store. How does it do? Oh, it's too acid. Now you got to go and get some cow manure, put on the thing, till it up, let it dry, go back another six weeks, and do it again. Oh, it's balanced, great. Now, our maid, she comes in. She said, "oh Wayne, we can't use this chemical here with this." I said, "Why" "Oh because it becomes toxic." And we know this. There are certain chemicals in the kitchen that we use that we can't mix with others, don't you agree. And they even say that on the label. Remember when you were in chemistry? They had these two jars, one of them was OK, one of them was OK, but the moment that you took a couple of drops from one to the other, remember the sparks that flew and all the gas and everything? If it happens in test tubes, it happens in your garden, and it happens in your kitchen, it happens in your stomach. Because this is nothing more than a mass of chemicals going on in the system. Massive amount of chemicals that's going on.

So, there are your three commandments of eating. Once again – desert the desserts, eat them before the meal, never after because this is where they are going to do the bulk of their digestion. Don't mix fruits and vegetables at the same meal – and keep your proteins and starches away from each other. Now what's a great holiday dinner?

Now all of you who are listening to this audio recording or watching this video series, and in this room here now, if you want to, let me have your name, full name, phone number, and e-mail address, and I will give you a year's subscription to our weekly E-zone, where once a week you'll get a free recipe and an empowering article and at the end of the month we give you an article. In the series that we've developed we have CDs that we produced with all of the ones, there is over a hundred, there's 100 recipe and 30 articles just on this CD. And so you can plug that in and you'll get them all. This is what you'll be receiving each week, the recipe and it's normally a $52.00 value per week, but the communication and all that we do, it's yours free, just for being here and being part of that two percent of the people who think logically for themselves. I really applaud you for being here because there are so few people who really think, so I appreciate that.

Now that you've got the three commandments of eating, who has a $20.00 on them? I need $20.00 here real quick, here's the man with the bucks. He says, no I've only got tens. Has anybody got 20 dollars on them real quick? Let me borrow that for a minute. Man I got me a poor group here. Now, I will give your twenty bucks back, so you're not out $20.00. I left my wallet in the room. I'm totally remiss. All right. Anybody can have this $20.00. Who wants it? Come on up and get it. Yeah, he says,

I want it back baby. Now. Ok. But wait a minute. All right, who wants the $20.00 now? Who would want it now? All right, I got some dirt, not much dirt. Who would want that $20.00 now?

OK. Now notice what you all did. Now there is a valuable lesson here. Sometimes in life we get dirt thrown on our faces. Sometimes we get slapped on the back. Stamped on. Sometimes we just get all wrinkled on the field like the Dickens. You know what I mean. And you don't feel like you're worth two cents. You get those down days. One word I want you to constantly remember when you get stressed out. When you get a feeling, tough thing, you're fed up. Just think of the word – cancel, cancel – I'm a special person. I have a unique quality. God never made a nobody. I'm special with unique qualities and just because you have all of these things pouring down on you, doesn't mean you're nobody. You're special with an unnegotiable self worth, just like this $20.00 bill that no matter how much dirt we threw on it, no matter how much I stamped on, no matter how much I crinkled it up, you wanted it. You know why? Because it has value. You have value. And if you'll eat good stuff, man, you'll always be tough. There's no doubt about it. You are special.

Here's a little poem to conclude this whole
Combine When You Dine seminar.

> When you hear that a person just died
>
> from a virus they found in his hide.
>
> Quite often you'll find
>
> that if you just learn how he dined
>
> that it should have been called
>
> suicide.

About the Author

Dr. Wayne "The Mango Man" Pickering, N.D., Th.D., Sc.M.

"THE AMBASSADOR for HEALTH"!

Author; Professional Speaker; Award Winning Triathlete & Double Nominee for The Healthy American Fitness Leader Award. His Prognosis was death at age 30. Now, at 72 years young he's a popular Nutritional Performance Coach, Lifestyle Management Consultant and a Disease Prevention Specialist who teaches people how to be the Healthiest Person ON the Planet and not the Wealthiest Person IN the Grave with a focus on Nutrition and a basic Philosophy, "If you want to be Tough you have to Eat Good Stuff" so you can get Older and Better and **not** Old and Bitter! He will also Show you how to Eat

More…Weigh Less…Sleep Better…Be Energized and Feel Terrific in 27 days, GUARANTEED!

Click here www.MangoManDiet.com for information if you would like our secrets on how to Eat More…Weigh Less…Sleep Better…Be Energized and Feel Terrific in 27 days, Guaranteed!

Contact Information

Published by:

The Center for Nutrition

1 Glowing Health Way

Box 26-3030

Daytona Beach, FL 32126

Phone: (866) MangoMan (626-4662)

Email: mangoman@WaynePickering.com

Copyright © 2011 by The Center for Nutrition. All rights reserved.

Legal Notice

If you obtained this report through any source but a purchase from http://www.waynepickering.com , you have purchased a pirated copy. Please contact mangoman@waynepickering.com to let us know where you got it.

varying international, federal, state and/or local laws or regulations. The purchaser or reader of this publication assumes responsibility for the use of these materials and information. Adherence to all applicable laws and regulations, including international, federal, state and local, governing professional licensing, business practices, advertising and all other aspects of doing business in the US, Canada or any other jurisdiction is the sole responsibility of the purchaser or reader. Neither the author nor the Publisher assume any responsibility or liability whatsoever on the behalf of any purchaser or reader of these materials.

Any perceived slight of specific people or organization is unintentional.